Hi5 Health Systems
presents

Strategic Health Solutions

Your simple plan to having it all!

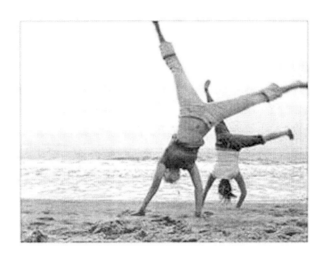

*"Give me the next 5 weeks
I'll give you the rest of your life"*

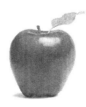

STRATEGIC HEALTH SOLUTION

Your simple plan to having it all!

Book design and layout by Perseus Design

ISBN

Printed in the United States of America

First Printing: 2011

IT'S YOUR TIME......

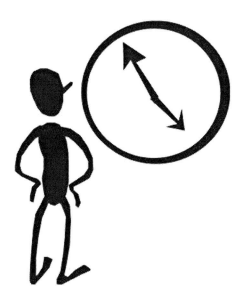

*Carpe diem! Rejoice while you are alive;
enjoy the day; live life to the fullest, make the
most of what you have. It could be later than
you think.*

Get started NOW!

Horace quote ~ ancient roman poet

Note To Reader

Here we are, *finally*! This book has been long time coming as a gift to all the wonderful people who have enjoyed Hi5 Produce and those of you excited about healthy living. From our first deliveries in 1996 until today, it has been an absolute pleasure serving you!

The idea of bringing fruit and vegetables came out of a desire to help people eat healthy on a consistent basis. We were active in teaching fitness and health, but the truth was, people needed more. We thought of the Hi5 Produce Delivery service like a nutrition personal trainer. We have come a long way, but our desire to help you make a healthy lifestyle easy, has not changed.

We honestly believe that when you eat food that energizes you, balanced with exercise and a great attitude, you will enjoy a more vibrant and happy life. Over the years, research has discovered so much in the area of healthy choices, but often times it gets over crowded in the variety of information out there. How are we supposed to know what to do and when? I am hoping the information in this book will guide you to exploring and discovering a healthy lifestyle that works for **you**.

Remember to keep everything in balance including adopting a healthy lifestyle. Don't let go of traditions and fun times. Try your best to follow the Hi5 Health System, but don't be hard on yourself if you mess up. Just smile and keep going. Give people around you grace if they are not where you are in the learning curve. Most importantly, HAVE FUN!

PS I am still learning too! If you see me at a burger joint, don't throw darts, it's probably my free day. :)

Denise T Locsin RN, Author, Speaker
Owner Hi5 Health Network
Hi5 Produce

Dedication

This book is dedicated to my best friend and the love of my life, my hubby, Danny. Thank you for inspiring me and believing in me since I was 16 years old.

I also dedicate this book to my four angels – Linnea, Isaiah, Ariana and Hannah. You are my "Why" in all I do.

I love you and I'm glad we are a team!

The Simple Health Solution
Table of Contents

Intro **17**

Chapter 1 How do you know when you are healthy? **21**

Chapter 2 Hi5 Health System **35**

Chapter 3 Fuel/Food **43**

Chapter 4 Fitness the 'Fountain of Youth' **61**

Chapter 5 Fun is an Attitude **71**

Chapter 6 Family and Friends – Let's rally the troops **79**

Chapter 7 Faith and Purpose **85**

Chapter 8 Making it Last **89**

Chapter 9 Beyond Foundation **97**

Chapter 10 Resources **103**

Acknowledgements

I always dreamt of the day that I could find a creative way to thank the amazing people who have blessed my life. How do I do that when the number of people I am thinking exceeds well over 200!! There is not enough room on this page to list you all by name, but I will do my best.

To my 79 nieces and nephews who I can say are my dearest friends. To my 9 brother-in-laws who make me feel safe and respected. To my 13 sister-in-laws who have become my best friends - I love you!

To my brothers Randy and Mark, you are such men of honor and I am so proud to be your sister. To Diane, my big sister, who always knows how to show love and speak incredible words of encouragement - I love you.

And to all my aunties, uncles and cousins who have touched my life with unconditional love, this book is for you.

To my church family, thank you for making me smile and especially Vanessa, Dawn, and Marlowe my spiritual sisters.

A special hug of gratitude to my dearest friend, Tricia, my true soul sister. My words cannot express my appreciation for all the years of support and friendship. I love you!

To my parents and in-laws who are the epitome of respect, family honor, love and everything that is virtuous in the world. For you, even acknowledgment in my book is not enough to tell you how much I love you. Thank you for being great parents.

To Chris who makes things run smooth-you rock! A special thank you to Becky who seems to make magic happen in the office-you are amazing. To Ann and Justin, I am honored to have you in my life-you make great things possible. To Fay who helps me dot my 'i's and cross the 't's – thank you!

To my Creator, to whom I give all the honor. I hope this book touches the lives it was meant to touch.

You're on this health journey, which road will you take?

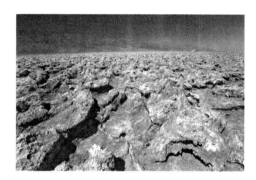

You can take the long way with roads that are bumpy and dry or . . . .

you can take the new freeway that is paved, and smooth.

I'll show you the road-map and you decide.

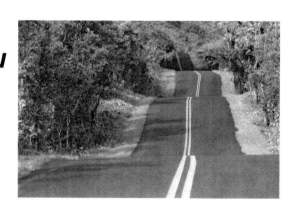

HOW TO USE THIS BOOK TO GET YOU WHERE YOU WANT TO GO

1. Read the book to get the big picture.

2. Get your calendar out and schedule your 5 weeks, including exercise times, free days, family time, etc.

3. Print the Hi5 Health System Grid and calendar tracker. This is KEY to success. It takes all the guess work out and keeps you on track.
(free download www.hi5healthnetwork.com)

4. Print Affirmations page and post where you can read frequently. You have to re-program the brain. (free download www.hi5-healthnetwork.com)

5. Create an Inspiration Poster and post it where everyone can see. Busyness and negative self talk will destroy your best efforts. Inspirational Poster will be a constant reminder of your "why". (www.hi5healthnetwork.com)

6. Start a health binder to collect information you find and keep a log of your meals for the 5 weeks. This will also be a great place to keep interesting articles, recipes, tips and other health info. Keeping everything in one place will make your life seem less hectic or overwhelming.

7. Gather resources that you will need for exercise, supplements, on-the-go meals, etc. Plan for the unexpected interruption by always being prepared.

8. Plan your meals and go shopping. You cannot break out of old habits until you make a conscious effort to establish new ones. See "must have" food staples in resource section.

9. Never look back. Smile and keep moving forward toward a healthier lifestyle even when life tries to throw you off course.

BEFORE WE BEGIN LET'S GET INTO THE RIGHT MINDSET.

10 WAYS TO STAY COMMITTED TO AN AWESOME AND HEALTHY FUTURE

1. I promise to read the book entirely with an open mind.

2. I promise to accept my mistakes as a growing and learning experience.

3. I promise to take responsibility for everything I put in my mouth.

4. I promise to move my body every day.

5. I promise to LAUGH.

6. I promise to SMILE.

7. I promise to have FUN on this journey.

8. I promise to stop negative self talk as soon as I notice it happening.

9. I promise to let guilt blow out the window and replace it with fascination.

10. I promise to believe that I deserve to be healthy!!

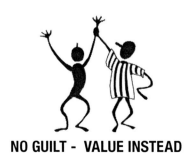

NO GUILT - VALUE INSTEAD

HERE WE GO.......

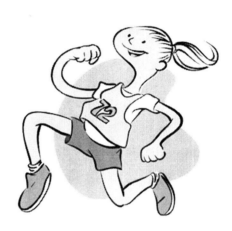

INTRO

After 22 years of exploring the mysteries of health, I have come to the conclusion that it is still a mystery. I have studied in the medical field and became a nurse only to discover health is a mystery there. I studied alternative philosophies and became a massage therapist and realized there are wide paradigms there too. Since then, my quest has been to find the commonalities in both. I began to look for a way to create a healthy foundation so that my body could withstand the bombardment of the toxins, viruses, germs, injury and stress we are constantly exposed to.

Having a healthy foundation would most importantly give me the springboard to rebound and heal quickly when I get sick or injured. It would be the foundation of a healthy lifestyle that I could maintain in busy times, stressful times and during plain ebbs and flows of life. It would be a lifestyle that would allow me to try other programs and diets without deviating from my core foundational routine. It had to allow me to live freely, enjoying barbecues, parties, vacations, and holidays *without guilt*.

I am excited to share with you my most amazing discoveries! Things that you might have already heard, but I am going to show you the most basic things you need to cover in establishing your health foundation. Once you establish your foundation, you can maintain this level of health and choose to be more aggressive when illness or injury strikes.

Some may find the pursuit of health so fascinating that you will want to explore more alternative philosophies and diets, and you will have a great foundation to work from. This can be a standalone program, but more importantly, it is a foundation to keep while you are on your health journey.

What are you looking for?

How about a system that is:

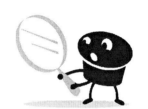

- Easy to follow
- Fun
- Filling
- Taste good
- Offer results you can see and feel!

Because I want you to get off to a solid start quickly, I offer a lot of information in a very simplified way. This book is about creating a lifestyle that you can live in without guilt, using simple action steps. For every idea, you will find a simple description for basic understanding. However, I encourage you to research further information from the material in the resource section of this book, on the internet and your local library.

For those of you like my husband who says:

"Just tell me what I need to do!"

This book has been written for you!

And for people like me who have to find the million whys behind it.

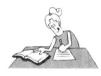 I offer resources in the back of the book.

Chapter 1:
How do you know when you are healthy?

What is your body telling you?

- *Your body speaks.*
- *What do the numbers say?*
- *Design your own health.*

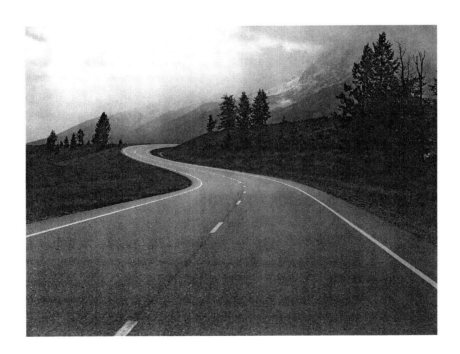

How do you know when you're there?

You know you are there when you think you are there and you just feel great. For most of us, that does not mean perfect health. Instead it is a balance between making healthy choices and taking responsibility for every outcome. For most of us, that is not a bikini body or running a marathon.

- Living healthy means you have **energy** to play with your children or grandchildren.

- Living healthy means having a **joy** that runs deep in your gut and allows you to take a deep breath.

- Living healthy means doing the day-to-day activities **without pain** or injury.

- Living healthy means having **mental clarity** in the midst of stress.

- Living healthy means playing in the rain **without getting sick.**

- Living healthy means getting sick and running to the health food store instead of the doctor to allow your **body to heal itself**.

Living healthy just feels good!
You will know when you are there!

Your Body Speaks to You!

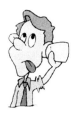
Your body is giving you messages everyday as to how it feels and what it wants in order to give you a great quality of life. The body craves to have balance free from harmful organisms, pain, injury, or out of whack hormones. It spends every moment fighting to keep you healthy. Every

sneeze or ache is the body shouting for assistance. All we have to do is listen and help out a little!

What do we have to do? First, just **NOTICE** that it is speaking to you. Then as you follow the Hi5 System, notice when the speaking quiets down. When you begin to recognize what helps and what doesn't, you can start taking control of your own health. Then, you can make choices consciously and know how to help your body get back on track.

Your Body's Reaction

Do you hate the word stress? The word itself conjures up thoughts of painful times, difficult people and overwhelm. The physiological response to stress, called "fight or flight", can be activated anytime our body must react to a threat caused by our environment or our thoughts. This is useful if the threat is real danger, but on a day to day basis it can cause long term damage.

This is the scenario inside your body when it reacts to stress as explained by Hans Selye, the first major researcher on stress:

When the body recognizes a problem, imagined or real, it causes the cerebral cortex, the thinking part of the brain to send an alarm signal to the hypothalamus (the main switch of the stress response, located in the mid brain). The hypothalamus then stimulates the Sympathetic Nervous System (SNS) to make a series of changes in your body. Your heart rate, blood volume and blood pressure go up. You start to perspire. Blood is directed away from the extremities and digestive system into the larger muscles that can help you fight or run. Your diaphragm and anus lock. Your adrenal glands start to secrete corticoids (adrenaline, epinephrine, norepinephrine) which inhibits digestion, reproduction, growth and tissue repair and the immune and inflammation response.

So you see, stress can be the primary cause of hypertension, heart disease, reproductive problems, loss of libido, asthma, diabetes, arthritis, muscle tension, fatigue, migraines, pre-mature aging, digestive problems such as ulcers, colitis, diarrhea or constipation and even cancer.

The good news is that every step in the Hi5 Health System is designed to aid your body in coping with stress and counter the negative effects. Living a healthy lifestyle is not about the right exercise or nutrition program or even the right therapy. Living a healthy lifestyle begins with creating a healthy mindset.

What is Healthy supposed to look like?

So, what is healthy actually supposed to look like? No one really knows! Yup, we have inclinations, but that is what makes health so much of a mystery. However, what we do know is really good. Every diet program, fitness program and new fad has its own idea and most of them actually work. How can this awesome vegetarian program and super fantastic high protein low carbohydrate diet both have great results and testimonials? They work because the body is fairly easy to please and it has more to do with the attitude and belief of the people in the program.

With that said, what do we know?

• Blood pressure should be 120/80

• Blood sugar less than 100mg/dl before eating. (70-125mg/dl)

• Resting Heart Rate between 50-100 beats/min. Well trained athletes will have much lower resting heart rate.

• Cholesterol Low LDL (bad cholesterol) and high HDL (good cholesterol) (HDL >60 considered protective against heart disease. HDL< 45 is considered increased risk of heart disease)

- pH will vary in different parts of body and different times. Blood pH 7.4

- Waist circumference ideally for women 28-33 inches and men 31-36 inches.

- Skin should be clear, radiant, even tone, and no blotches.

- Energy level should be steady and vibrant during normal waking hours

- Weight should be within range for height and weight according to Body Mass Index BMI

- Hormones within normal ranges per blood or saliva test.

- Stress level should be low

- Sleep at least 7 hours per night

- Attitude should be joyful and optimistic all the time (hee hee that is what I tell my kids!!)

- Shoe size should be .... are we getting out of hand? Yes!!!! Don't get paranoid, obsessive or fanatic of all the should'ves. These are just baselines in a perfect world. Can we aim for it? Oh yeah, why not see what your body can do!

Reality Please!

Ok, so where do we start?

First thing you want to do is get your baselines recorded on your Hi5 Health Grid so you can get them out of the way. I'd like to say don't worry about them at all but if you don't get some baselines, you will never know how you progressed or learn how to hear your body. It's also great motivation and gives you bragging rights.

How do you know when you are healthy?

Hi5   Action Steps

- Gather all your **measurements and record them** on the Hi5 Health System Grid. Don't analyze them or feel down about your results, just record and be on your merry way.

- One huge special request: Take a **before photo**. No other way! We humans are very visual and this will be great motivation, as well as help you notice changes. Here's an idea if you are too shy to ask for assistance: Put your bathing suit on and use a camera with a timer or take a photo using your camera phone and email it to yourself. If that is difficult, you can take a photo of your reflection in the mirror.

- Start a **Healthy Living binder** and add all your baselines to your binder.

How do you know when you are healthy?

What does healthy look like to you?

_____

_____

_____

_____

What do you want your health to look like?

_____

_____

_____

_____

Can you see that vision in your mind? Begin with the end in mind. Vision is essential.

_____

_____

The Science Behind It, in my Unscientific Way

B/P - Blood pressure tells you how hard your heart is working to pump throughout your body. The top number represents how hard your heart is working at time of contraction. The bottom number represents how hard your heart is working at time of relaxation. For that reason, the bottom number is significantly important in telling us how your heart is working at rest.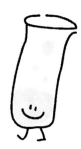

Blood Sugar - Blood sugar levels tell you how much sugar is floating around and not being used in the cell. Free floating sugar causes things to get rotten and is bad for internal environment. Sugar is a key contributor to inflammation, aging, low immune system, pain in joints and fatigue.

Heart Rate - This tells you how many times per minute your heart contracts and relaxes. Obviously your heart rate will go up during exercise, but should go back down at a good rate when you stop exercising. Notice how your heart rate increases during stress.

Cholesterol - Although your cholesterol levels are important to monitor, it is not the cause of heart disease. In reality HDL actually protects the heart by cleaning out LDL stuck on arterial walls. Triglycerides are a major player in the dance between HDL (good) and LDL (bad). Too much triglycerides cause decrease in HDL and increase in LDL. Triglycerides come from, you guessed it, sugar and processed foods.

pH - Our body is in constant state of acid/base balance. Foods that cause our body to be more acidic require alkalotic rich foods to balance pH. A constant state of acidosis has shown to contribute to chronic inflammation. Some food that balance our pH and create a healthy internal ecosystem include vegetables especially greens, sauerkraut, lemons and lime.

Waist - Measured at the smallest point of the waist below the ribs. Fat that you can see around the waist is called subcutaneous fat. The more dangerous fat is around the organs called visceral fat which is not visible. Waist measurement is a good indicator of visceral and subcutaneous fat.

Skin – It's the largest organ in the body and its function is to excrete, protect and insulate. Your skin is a good indicator of what is going on inside your body. Skin is affected by stress, toxicity, sugar, lack of sleep, hydration and malnourishment. Since your skin is an organ that feeds directly to the blood stream – rule of thumb- if you can't eat it, don't put it on your skin.

Energy – Low energy is normal when you are tired from lack of sleep or intense work, but it becomes unusual when you wake up feeling tired or spend most of your waking hours drained. This may be dehydration, depression, lack of nutrients, or some other underlying cause. Unfortunately, it is not easy to pinpoint the cause. Once you begin to consistently make healthy choices, you will feel your level of energy soar.

Weight - Body Mass Index BMI is a guide to measure body fat based on height and weight. BMI is used as a guide. Since it only considers height and weight, there is no distinction between fat tissue or muscle. For that reason, many well trained athletes have a high BMI due to muscle tissue. Because of all the unique variables, BMI should only be used as an indicator to where we generally fall and to notice changes.
BMI = (weight divided by height squared) x 703.
Below 18.5 underweight
18.5 – 24.9 normal weight
25 – 29.9 overweight
30 above obese

Hormones- Hormones are chemicals that travel to organs in the body to coordinate sophisticated processes such as growth, metabolism, fertility and a host of other body functions. They have influences over immune system and even mood and behavior. For an in-depth look at delicate balance of hormones and their importance, read Hormone Balance Made Simple by John Lee MD and his other amazing books on hormone balance.

Stress – Periodically, stress is a normal part of life. Stress becomes a physiological problem when it is chronic state and the body doesn't get a rest. Stress has one of the most toxic effects on your body. In a nut shell, a chronic levels of stress on the body is like a slow suicide.

Sleep - Research has shown that people who sleep less than 7-8 hrs per night have higher incident of weight gain and stress. Lack of sleep becomes an uphill battle.

Attitude - Our attitude or how we interpret an event is completely voluntary therefore; the physiological side affect is voluntary. If we choose a negative attitude such as anger, frustration, sadness or resentment, our body responds with negative chemical reactions. These chemical reactions mess up our immune system, hormones, mental state, etc. The flip side is: a positive attitude like happiness, gratitude, forgiveness and love, cause the body to release hormones that strengthen our immune system, balance hormones and decrease inflammation.

Design your own health

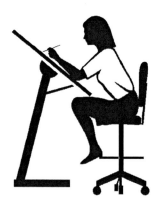

Imagine what results you want to see and write it on the Health Grid. The physical act of writing something down causes the subconscious to think it is real and will strive to fulfill the vision.

How do you know when you are healthy?

Hi5 Action steps:

* List the baseline parameters that you want to see.

* Be realistic but stretch yourself and watch what happens.

Note: It is important to get a physical before beginning any exercise program. You can obtain much of the baseline information from your physical.

	Baselines	**Vision**
B/P		
HR Rest & Exercise		
Bl Sugar		
Waist circumference		
BMI		
Weight		
How do you feel?		
What are your areas of concern?		
photo		

How do you know when you are healthy?

Straight talk with Denise:

Gathering your baselines numbers seems cumbersome, but it is very important. Don't dwell on the results. You are creating a lifestyle, not following a strict regime. Spend some time visualizing what you want your health to look like. Describe your vision on your Hi5 Health Grid so you can stay focused. Once you have imagined your results and have written it down your subconscious does everything it can to make it reality.

Have fun imagining how to get the results you want.

Chapter 2:
Hi5 Health System

Blueprint to building your strong foundation

The roadmap will get you there. The Hi5 Health System
The principles are keys to live by. The Hi5 Principles
The philosophy is a way of believing to get the outcome you desire.
The Hi5 Philosophy
The right mindset is a way to think so you always stay on track.
The Hi5 Mindset

Build your health foundation so strong that no California earthquake
will knock you down!

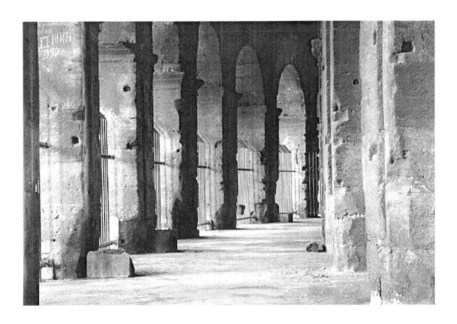

Hi5 Health System

The Hi5 Health System is a **tool** for you to use to help you grow a strong, resilient and solid foundation. It is a **roadmap** to follow as you progress on this health journey. The main premise is that if you establish a healthy foundation, you will experience fewer colds and flues, have more energy, sleep better, get to your ideal weight naturally, maintain a better mood, effortlessly move through activities of your day and give your body a fighting chance to prevent serious diseases. It does not mean that you will never get sick, stress out, lose your patience, get tired, or stub your toe. What it means is that you will improve the **QUALITY** of your life by leaps and bounds and **REBOUND** quicker if illness or disease does strike.

Hi5 Health System
The Power of "5"

- 5 Piers

- 5 Days per Week

- 5 Weeks

Focus on 5 areas of your life for 5 days per week for 5 weeks. They say if you do anything for 21 days it will become a habit in your life. We will simply space it out and put a few extra days for back up. There are 5 target areas in life that determine the quality of your every day.

This chapter reviews the Hi5 Health System. Once you follow the Hi5 Health System and use the Hi5 Health Grid, all the principles, philosophies and mindset will make sense and be easy to implement. REMEMBER the key to your success is using the Hi5 Health Grid. The Hi5 Health Grid takes all the confusion away. It is like an architect who invests the time to draw up blueprints to a house. A good set of blueprints to a house helps you see what the house will look like when it is done and what steps need to be done to get there. The blueprint lays out the building of the home into manageable steps. During the construction of a house, if schedule has interruptions or delays, it is easy to pick up the blueprint and begin right where they left off. If the interruption caused a set back or change, the contractor simply adjusts and gets right back on track according to the plan. That is exactly how the Hi5 Health Grid works!

Choose any five days per week to think about these target areas and then enjoy two days where you don't even think about it. Two days where you are free to eat junk, guzzle down soda, enjoy road rage, slump on the sofa all day, yell at the kids, and have a meltdown. Yup, live your old way to the fullest! Enjoy! All you have to do is describe how you feel the day after. No guilt at all, just make a mental note each week. The great thing about having two free days is that if you go off track during the week, you can make it a free day and you still have another free day for the weekend.

Many programs recommend only one free day, however, I found that the idea of gorging on the one free day became a primary focus. Remember this is a lifestyle, therefore, it must be a routine you can live within. If later on in your journey you decide to try a program that gives one free day, or no free days, it will be that much easier for you.

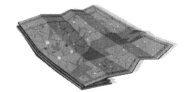

Hi5 Principles

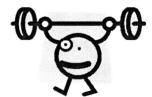

- Strengthen the Cells

- Good In

- Bad Out

Does that sound too simple? It isn't when you consider that every choice we make either makes our cells stronger or weaker. Since our cells determine how our body and mind function, if we take care of our cells they'll take better care of us. That means; aim for putting good stuff in so our cells do the job well. Be conscious of getting the bad stuff out via sweat, poop, respiration, and urine. By recognizing how junk is expelled from our body, we can even be more aggressive after we have junked out. Even if you ate like a saint, you would still have junk that the body has to expel daily from the byproduct the cells create after doing their job. Just sitting on the sofa all day creates byproduct that has to come out, so make it priority.

Hi5 Philosophy

1. Balanced internal **ecosystem** means that destructive organisms cannot grow out of control.

2. Establish an efficient **sewage system** so garbage goes out (disposal) and nutrients are absorbed and utilized correctly (recycle).

3. Everything we do either **strengthens our cells** or weakens them and that determines our quality of life.

4. Attitude is everything. Wherever you place your thoughts is where you will go.

Hi5 Mindset

Really, all this health stuff is a **choice** based on the conversation you are having in your head.

- A healthy mindset means being completely aware of what you eat and how it affects your body and making the best food choices for your health.

- A healthy mindset means you are compelled to exercise daily because you value your body, your energy, and your future.

- A healthy mindset means discovering ways to let go of stress and negative emotions because you understand its toxic damage.

- Finally, a healthy mindset means you are excited about life (no matter the circumstances) and the daily discovery of new things.

The 5 Piered Foundation:

Pier holes are used to make really strong concrete foundations, so for our purposes we are going to make a 5 pier hole foundation. When we address these 5 areas we create a super strong foundation.

The 5 areas include:

- Fuel/ Food
- Fitness
- Fun
- Family
- Faith

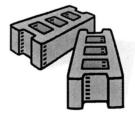

Straight talk with Denise:

You can do this! It may seem overwhelming at times but relax, enjoy the process and let the system do it for you. The secret to making all these steps simple and automatic is in the Hi5 Health Grid. By knowing what you are going to do in advance on a daily basis, makes it easy to prepare and implement.

Remember, you deserve to feel healthy. So, go print the Hi5 Health Grid right NOW! Begin NOW! Fill out the information that you can and begin taking control of your health. Print a few and post them where you can see them often. Print them on 8 ½ x 11 paper or larger to really make a big impact.

Find downloadable copy of Hi5 Health Grid at www.hi5health-network.com

Hi5 Health System

FOOD & FUEL
- Cut meal size in 1/2
- Choose low glycemic foods
- No calorie counting
- Balance pH & alkalotic foods
- Photo each meal

Warning! Highly processed white bread, white pasta, artificial sweeteners, soft drinks and high fructose corn syrup ARE TOXIC!

~ Daily Routine ~

- VitMin
- EFA
- Probiotics
- Enzyme
- Fiber
- Fruit
- H2O
- High Nutrient drink

MEALS: 5 meals per day

- High Nutrient drink
- Breakfast
- Snack
- Lunch
- Snack
- Dinner

Energy Foods that fuel

* Back-up plan!!
* Triple Threat: 60/60 lunges, 60 p/u, 100 abs

www.hi5healthnetwork.com

FITNESS!

Exercise is a gift! Proven to decrease all forms of disease, slow down the aging process, eliminate depression, balance hormones and improve all aspects of life!

What do you like to do?

Plan ahead, keep it simple & be consistent. 10-25 min/day.

- Week 1:
- Week 2:
- Week 3:
- Week 4:
- Week 5:

Family
Your Why!!

Everyone is starving for attention. Give it freely. Tell them daily!

List who or allow photo

What will you do?

- Wk1
- Wk2
- Wk3
- Wk4
- Wk5

FUN!
Be Optimistic!

Hang out with positive people!

What will you do for fun this week?

Faith

Your life has   Find the peace to   Ask for your

What will you do this week to grow your faith?

Chapter 3:
Fuel, Food or Folly?

What is your biggest food challenge? Is it not knowing what to eat or how to prepare it? Or feeling hungry all the time? Or do you think what you eat has no influence on your health?

Let's imagine for a moment that everything you eat is what you are made of tomorrow. Let's imagine that you always felt nutritionally content and you eat for enjoyment and energy. Let's imagine that what you eat and how to prepare it is easy and automatic.

My body is a temple where junk food goes to worship.
unknown author

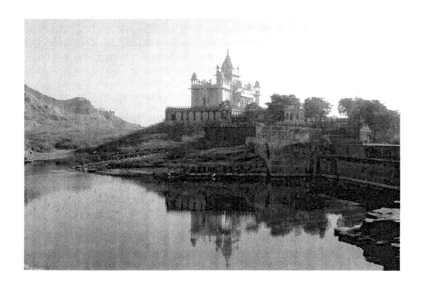

Fuel/ Food

Food is awesome!

Eating is one of the greatest pleasures in life. Food has power to heal the body, nurture relationships, bond families, soothe the soul, give us abundant energy and make everything more fun. Food is your greatest commodity. Use it wisely and you will thrive.

I think the biggest challenge we have with poor nutrition is too many choices and not knowing their affect on our bodies. In our area we had the Body World Exhibit, where you were able to see real organs from donors who had offered their bodies to science. The reality hits you when you see a real human's healthy lung next to a smoker's lung.

We talk about fat loss as if it is an esthetic goal, a goal that will make us look good in shorts or impress someone else. We often want to accomplish a weight goal because we want to look like some ideal image we created in our heads or seen on TV. Again, reality sends chills down your back when you see a cross section of an obese adult and realize how the fat surrounds and suffocates the heart, the liver and every organ in the body. It makes sense that the liver is struggling to detox the body. It makes sense that we have shortness of breath. It makes sense that we have poor blood circulation. It all begins to make sense when you see it in real life!

So, when you think about food, think of it as fuel that allows your body to flourish. It's not a diet of deprivation, but an eating style that will make you feel satisfied and alive.

Conscious eating

Do you remember what it was like, learning how to drive a car? It seemed impossible to think about every pedal, the speed limit, the rules, knowing where you were going, looking in the side mirror, rear view mirror, turning your head and putting your blinkers on, all at the same time. That's assuming you remembered to check the gas, fasten your seat belt, and bring your driver's license. Ughhhh!! way too much to think about! But you did it (well most of us). That is what it's like learning a new eating style. Overwhelming at first, but eventually it becomes second nature.

It begins with looking at your food. Actually looking at each bite and casually thinking of how it's going to nourish your cells or hurt them. It is ok either way, because it is your choice. Accept the choice you make and move on. Do this every time and you will begin to notice how certain foods change your mood, and how they make you feel, physically. It is that awareness that will move you toward healthy choices.

Since we prepare meals and eat so subconsciously and habitual, we need to keep a food photo diary. Get in the habit of taking a picture of everything that goes into your mouth during your 5 weeks. Most of us have camera-phones that make it really easy to snap a quick shot.

Hi5 Action step:

- **Photo** of everything you eat for these 5 weeks to teach you to be conscious of what you eat. This is a key step toward awareness and conscious eating.

- Add the pictures to your **health binder**

No Calorie Counting

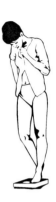

Talk about taking all the fun out of eating. Counting calories is not a way to live anyway. Simply remember that the biggest calorie contributors are soft drinks, fruit juice, white bread, white pasta, high fructose corn syrup, highly processed foods, and of course sweets. If you choose to incorporate these in your diet, they WILL sabotage any healthy lifestyle goals. Instead, follow these basic rules:

Hi5 Action steps:

- Drink a glass of water with lemon prior to eating your meal. You will feel fuller and it will start the digestive process in preparation for food that is on its way.

- Start all your meals with salad or other abundance of veggies. The high fiber will satisfy the hunger faster and jump start the digesting process.

- Enjoy a grapefruit or take an enzyme supplement before eating to make digestion smooth.

- Eat slowly to give the brain time to recognize that you are eating and send signals that tell the body to release a hormone called leptin that tells your body that you are nutritionally satisfied and it's ok to stop eating.

- Don't watch TV or read while eating, because you will go into subconscious mode and habitual eating and end up over eating.

- Eat smaller portions. If you have smaller portions and you eat slower, your body will be just as satisfied as if you had eaten double the meal. You can always save the rest for the next snack meal. This will help keep sugar level steady.

- Most importantly, be ok with not finishing your meal. Stop when satisfied, not when stuffed or when plate is empty. This can be emotionally challenging for some people, but just tell yourself you can eat it later.

- Chew! Chew 27 times before swallowing. Not an easy thing to do, but you get the idea!

Glycemic Index

The Glycemic Index was created to give each food a value to show how it affects the insulin spikes in our blood stream. The extremes of the spectrum include table sugar at the top with a value of 100 and proteins at the low with a value of zero. There have been some adjustments to the original index to now look at how the food affects you once in the body. This is important because originally fruit had a high glycemic index, but under the glycemic load, fruit has a much smaller number.

The importance of the Glycemic Load is that it teaches us how foods affect our insulin levels. Insulin in our blood stream holds onto fat. Losing weight then becomes an impossible battle when we are eating a diet that keeps our insulin levels at a constant high or spikes. Like swimming upstream with a heavy dumbbell tied to your foot. Keep your insulin levels low and even for weight loss.

Keep it simple choose vegetables as your carbohydrate at each meal! Charts and lists are often cumbersome to follow so make it simple by choosing an abundance of vegetables. If you desire to eat a starchy carbohydrate, choose as close to natural as possible, such as whole grain breads or pastas or brown rice, but in small portions. When it comes to starchy carbohydrates, think small portions and eat real slow to allow the sugar to enter the cells and trigger a hormone reaction that tells your body that you are full.

Hi5 Action steps:

• Choose foods that have a low glycemic load such as protein, vegetables, fruit and oatmeal. If you do eat foods with a high glycemic load, you can balance it out with foods that are low glycemic to give you a balanced insulin increase.

• Post a list of low glycemic foods as a reference on your fridge to make it easy to know what to eat. Download free list www.hi5-healthnetwork.com

• Avoid highly processed foods because they will definitely spike your insulin levels with all hidden sugars like high fructose corn syrup and other sweeteners.

• Do not substitute sugar with artificial sweeteners such as aspartame, saccharin, sucralose (splenda) despite their small affect on insulin levels. The toxic damage they have at the cellular level is far more damaging over time. This is one of the most destructive things that you can do to your body and the affects last for years.

pH

One of the Hi5 philosophies is to create a strong internal ecosystem so bad organisms cannot grow or take over. Here is where it begins to make sense. Our body has a pH that tends to be more alkalotic 7.4 and when we do things that cause our body to be acidic, we create a breeding ground for foreign organisms to flourish like viruses, bacteria, fungus, parasites and even worms to live. When this happens our bodies immune system goes into overdrive creating inflammation to try to fix the problem. Unfortunately, if we stay in a constant acidic state, inflammation doesn't stop and the inflammation itself wears down our body.

How do we get acidic? Sugar, stress, obesity, allergens (pollen, gluten etc.), smoking, pesticides, coffee, chemicals, high carbohydrates diet, lack of sleep, and the junk food we are so familiar with. Don't worry; there are easy things to do to dim the effects.

Hi5 Action steps:

- Take Omega 3 Essential Fatty Acids everyday!

- Lemon water first thing upon rising. We wake up in an acidic state and lemon water gets you closer to the correct alkalosis state.

- Did I mention avoid sugar? Sugar throws your body into an acidic state, creates inflammation and feeds organisms. So, avoid sugar as much as possible.

- Visit the ocean to benefit from its negative ions in the air. The healing benefits of the negative ions from the crashing waves can combat some of our worst offenses.

- Drink lots for water. You have heard it before so I am just reminding you.

- Apple cider vinegar (Braggs brand) I use 2 caps full to 3 oz of water. I actually hate the taste, so often I just gargle and spit. When I do drink it I dilute it even more.

- Eat a lot of fruits and vegetables which are alkaline.

Vitamins and Minerals

It's funny how we always say vitamins and minerals together like 'bread and butter' or 'MasterCard and Visa' when actually, they are very different.

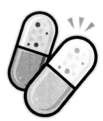

Vitamins assist with communication in the cell. When specific vitamins are missing, certain functions can't happen or happen incorrectly.

Minerals perform different activities in the body to help transfer energy to carry out specific functions. We are often fatigued if we do not get enough minerals on a daily basis.

In a perfect world, you could get all the necessary vitamins and minerals from the foods we eat, but reality doesn't allow us to eat perfectly. Therefore, vitamin and mineral supplements are vital in combination with nutrient rich foods like vegetables and fruit.

Hi5 Action Steps:

- Find a good vitamin and mineral supplement from a reputable company or a reputable store like Whole Foods.

- Start juicing! Juicing is a great way to extract nutrients and water from vegetables and fruit. Search the internet for great juicing recipes.

Enzymes

This is literally the key to restoring pH balance, proper digestion and absorption of nutrients. Also a great way to help the pancreas since it produces less enzymes as we age. Try supplementing your diet and eating more raw vegetables and fruit. Notice how your digestive system feels over time after incorporating digestive enzymes to your supplements.

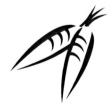

Hi5 Action steps:

* Make sure to get your enzymes in before each meal via supplement.

* Eat 1/2 grapefruit before meals.

* Eat raw vegetables at each sitting to provide an abundance of food enzymes.

Fruit

It goes without saying, fruit is the hero in making this whole process of healthy lifestyle pleasurable. With fruit you get nutrients to feed the cells, water that tastes great, fiber to curb our hunger, sugar that doesn't spike our insulin levels, no preparation time, elegantly packaged in array of colors, variety of intense flavors that keep us from getting bored, great shelf life, easy to get and the list goes on. You see why fruit can be your hero too, on this health journey!

Action Steps:

* Eat fruit daily as an appetite suppressor, added nutrients, natural energy and more fiber.

* Enjoy your fruit between meals, not with your meals.

Probiotics

Good bacteria have a very protective job in our digestive system. We must replenish our good bacteria on a consistent basis. Probiotics protect by inhibiting the overgrowth of bad organisms. Probiotics are the main players in creating a healthy internal ecosystem in your body. When you have a lot of good bacteria in your gut, the body doesn't have to work so hard to fight foreign organisms and it can use its energy on other tasks.

Hi5 Action Steps:

- Supplement with a good probiotic.

- Eat fermented foods like sauerkraut, kimchee, kephur and yogurt as an add on to your meals.

Essential Fatty Acids

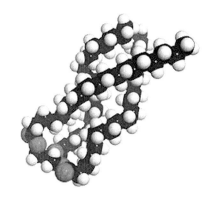

Keeping it simple. Think about omega 3 essential fatty acids this way: Low omega 3 essential fatty acids = brittle and inflamed vs high omega 3 essential fatty acids= subtle and elasticity at every tissue in the body including the brain.

EFA's are used to make strong cell membranes. If you do not have enough EFA on board, the body will use unhealthy fats from donuts, french fries or white bread to make weak cell membranes. These weak cells will break easy, age easy and not be able to ward off invaders like free radicals. Free radicals are harmful molecules that damage and attack cells. Antioxidants like Vit C, Vit D etc., attack the free radicals to stop the attack on the cell membranes. EFA's make the cell membranes strong and resilient.

Although there is not a standard dosage recommendation, EFAs are safe at low or high amounts. I have found better results in amounts greater than 2 grams. Make sure your supplement includes DHA and EPA which is great for brain health.

Hi5 **Action steps:**

- Supplement with essential fatty acids everyday is crucial for a strong foundation!

Fiber

A food that has no nutritional value other than keeping an efficient sewage system, ridding our body of toxins and helping us feel full thus preventing cancer and improving weight loss. Pretty important don't you think? Fiber is vital to good health and easy to get if you eat a diet high in fruits, vegetables and legumes. But in reality, we don't always get an abundance of fruits, vegetables and legumes on a daily basis so it's a good idea to supplement also. A good fiber supplement with no taste is easy to mix in protein shakes or other drinks.

Hi5 **Action Steps:**

- Strive to get 24 grams of fiber per day. Difficult to do especially for us people on the go, which is why you want to find a good fiber supplement.

- Make sure you drink plenty of water when increasing fiber in your diet.

- Include veggies with each meal.

- Choose fruit or veggies for snacks.

Water

You have probably heard it said that the body is 70% water or some other number like that, but what is that supposed to mean? Basically, we are moist inside like a snail. As a child, the kids in the neighborhood

thought it was so funny to pour salt on snails
and watch them shrivel and die. I was ter-
rified of snails so I hated the whole thing.
We are similar in that much of what we are
exposed is pulling water from our body and
we need to replenish daily to prevent dehy-
dration and shriveling up.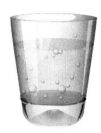

If you are drinking less than 64 oz or 8 glasses of water per day
chances are you are dehydrated. Often overeating is caused by dehydration. Soda, juices and coffee don't count.

Hi5 Action steps:

- Shoot for minimum 8 glasses of water, but more is better.

- Get a water purifier or reverse osmosis.

5 Small Meals per day

This does not mean 5 feasts per day because the scale would
surely sky rocket. The idea of the 5 small meals spaced over the day
is to trick the body into never going into starvation mode, which
will cause it to hold fat. If the body thinks we are depriving it of
food, it will hold onto what it already has and what comes in. In
addition, it keeps your blood sugar level so your energy level stays
consistent. Finally, adopting the idea of 5 meals per day will mentally keep you satisfied.

When planning your meals include a protein, fat and carbohydrate
(primarily vegetable carbohydrate) at each meal. Think wholesome
foods that come as natural as possible. The more processed the food
the harder it is for your body to utilize it for fuel and it becomes dangerous instead of helpful. Because you will be eating 5 meals per day
you can easily cut your portion sizes in half and still feel completely

satisfied. In addition, once you feed your body the nutrients it needs from the supplements, your cells won't be starving therefore, you will lose the need to overeat.

Also, if you find yourself hungry between meals drink a glass of water, take a walk, eat a protein or snack on carrots or some other vegetable.

Hi5 Action steps:

- Plan ahead. This can be elaborate or very simple. Use your Hi5 Health Grid to list great meal ideas.

- Make one or even two meals the same every day as to eliminate spontaneous eating. I always have oatmeal in the morning with almonds and blueberries and usually a salad with protein of some sort for lunch.

- Have a protein, carbohydrate in form of veggies and fat, at every meal. Slowly decrease your quantity of complex carbohydrates like bread, rice and pasta.

- If you feel hungry at other times, drink water or eat another fruit.

- Protein - Proteins are important building blocks for the body, weight loss, hormone production, healing tissues and provide a feeling of being nutritionally satisfied.

- Fats are an essential part of life. Good sources of fat are olive oil, avocados, seeds, nuts, fish, coconut oil, flaxseed. Research has found supplementing with Omega3 Essential Fatty Acids has proven to have great benefit to disease prevention, fat loss, anti aging, and mental clarity.

- Carbohydrates - Carbohydrates are important as a quick energy but what you don't use will have to be stored as fat. Focus on eliminating processed carbohydrates (cookies, white bread, pasta, crackers, chips) and replacing them with complex carbohydrates (vegetables, whole grain foods, oatmeal, quinoa).

Here is where a big problem lies in the traditional American diet. Manufactures have been loading the highly processed foods with high fructose corn syrup and other fillers that are proving to have catastrophic affects. High Fructose Corn Syrup is cheap and easy to manufacture from corn, but in high amounts, we are seeing serious problems to health. Keep your ears open to this topic. I think we will hear more and more about the long term detrimental effects.

Hi5 Action Steps:

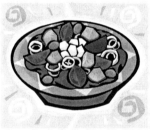

- Include lean protein with each meal: meat, chicken, fish, nuts, eggs and legumes.

- Don't waste your health on empty calories like white bread, white pasta, white crackers, and highly processed foods. If you choose to do that, it will accumulate over time.

- Get your carbs from vegetables and in small portions whole grains, brown rice, quinoa and oatmeal.

- Get your good fats from supplements, avocados, salmon, sardines, olive oil, and coconut oil.

- Cut portion sizes in half. If you are eating half the amount, but eating slowly and taking supplements, you will feel nutritionally satisfied.

What meals can you choose for breakfast?

_____

_____

What meals can you choose for lunch?

_____

_____

What meals can you choose for dinner?

_____

_____

What healthy snack options can you have available?

_____

_____

What are your biggest obstacles to choosing healthy foods?

_____

_____

Create your daily routine:

What vitamin and mineral supplement will you use? Where will you get it? _____

_____

_____

What Essential Fatty Acid will you take? How many grams per day will you take? _____

_____

_____

What ways will you get your probiotics? _____
_____
_____

What enzymes will you take and how often? _____
_____
_____

How will you get your 24 grams of fiber each day?
_____
_____
_____

What fruits do you like to eat? _____
_____
_____

Do you like water? How much will you drink per day?
Do you have a special to go container for your water?
_____
_____
_____

What high nutrient drink will you incorporate into your
diet? (juicing, protein, fiber, green drinks, coconut water etc.) _____
_____
_____

Straight talk with Denise

When it comes to food, don't expect perfection. I once tried to be a vegetarian because I thought it would give me more energy. I was 22 and didn't know how to cook, so I lived on peanut butter and jelly sandwiches and bean burritos. That didn't work and my energy plummeted. I have learned how to have fun with food and use it to accomplish what I want.

Foods that are alive provide lots of enzymes, vitamins, minerals and fiber so try to eat as much live food as possible and you will feel alive. The more it's cooked or altered, the less the nutritional value, with the exception of meat, chicken and fish, which should be cooked.

One of the great things about taking supplements is that you are no longer starving nutritionally, therefore you won't need to gorge. You will learn to eat for fuel and pleasure.

Chapter 4:
Fitness the Fountain of Youth

Convince Me!!

- *Minimum requirement*
- *Trick yourself*
- *What to expect*
- *What to choose*

If it wasn't for dogs, some people would never go for a walk!

The older you get, the tougher it is to lose weight because by then, your body and your fat are really good friends.

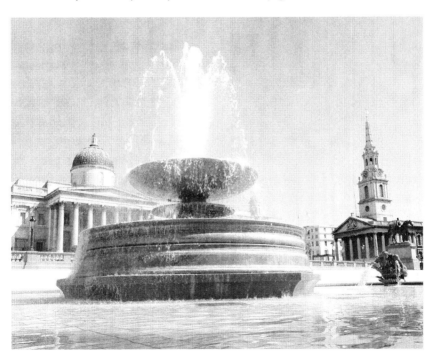

Fitness / Fountain of Youth

Can I just say I have never really liked exercising? There, I said it! I feel much better now. It seemed silly to spend an hour in the gym, wandering around, wondering what to do, and maybe run on a treadmill for 30 minutes followed by several different machines that I did not know how to use. I did find it easier to stay committed to scheduled fitness classes or personal training. However, once the class ended or my schedule changed, I was off an exercise routine again.

Everything changed for me when I discovered interval training for short periods of time. Short periods of time with great results!

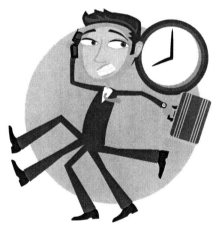

Convince Me of the Benefits because I don't have time!

The greatest convincing I ever got was when someone told me **'if there was ever a fountain of youth, it is exercise'**. Ok let me rethink this exercise thing. All these years I have been exercising to prep for summer attire. I know the health benefits of lowering blood pressure, strengthen the heart, decrease stress etc, but sometimes it just isn't enough motivation.

A study done on cool little fit mice and couch potato mice showed interesting results. The researchers forced one group of mice to exercise for 40 minutes three times per day, while the other mice were kept sedentary.

After several months the fit mice looked younger and had sleek coats with the effects of aging virtually non-existent in any of their organs. The sedentary mice however, were graying, slow-moving, socially isolated, mental deterioration, organ failure and less fertile.

The researchers believe the key is in the mitochondria of the cell. Mitochondria in the cells are where metabolism takes place, therefore it is known as the 'power house'. Healthy abundant mitochondria equals energy, youthfulness and slowing the aging process.

Another motivating benefit is that muscles are actually fat burning machines that burn fat tissue throughout the day. That is what I call residual effect. No muscle=no fat burning, it's that simple!

Focus on the core muscles which are around the waist. The mid section is where we hide the dangerous fat around the organs. Sorry skinny people, you are not off the hook from exercising if you want to stay young.

Minimum needed to get benefits

Imagine you set your timer for 25 minutes, blast your music, start your interval timer, look up at the wall for the exercises you can do, and go. That's it. Keep going till the 25 minute timer goes off, cool down and you are done. Of course you want to get a 2 to 5 minute warm up in the beginning and a 2 to 5 minute cool down at the end, which can include your stretching.

My interval timer is set for 50 seconds on and 10 second rest but you want to begin where you are comfortable. By alternating short intense exercise sessions with short rest, you burn more fat calories, strengthen the heart, and have greater fat loss hours after you are done exercising. The traditional aerobic exercising where you huff and puff but can still keep on a conversation, has proven to be ineffective at fat loss and muscle tone.

If you are new to exercising or are out of shape, spend the first week and up to 4 weeks getting your body adjusted to moving. Start by walking then progress to interval training. Once you are ready, incorporate 10 minutes of interval training and then progress from there. It goes without saying to get a physical prior to beginning any exercise program.*

Trick Yourself

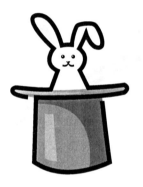

I gotta tell you, interval training in itself, is a big trick because it is so automated and short that before you know it, it is over. No time to dread it or be interrupted. Blasting your upbeat music is a trick because you can't hear the negative or distracting thoughts in your head. My favorite is an upbeat funky gospel CD that not only makes me move but keeps me positive too.

Try to plan your exercising in the morning because it is hard to skip out if you have already done it. Plus you have probably had caffeine which will give you an energy boost to move. If you need to eat prior, have a protein shake 30 minutes before for fuel. Make a list of all the possible exercises that you can do and post them on the wall where you like to exercise so it is available at all times. This way you do not have to waste time wondering.

---

* See the list of a few exercises to choose in the resource section in the back of the book

What to expect

- Yes, you will be **sore but not forever**. Once you build enough mito-chondria in the cells you will no longer get sore as frequently. Don't skip your workout just because you are sore. Exercising through it will help get rid of the lactic acid and get rid of the pain faster.

- Ladies, No, you won't bulk up like massive man body builder. I recommend you alternate with Yoga or Pilates anyway to give you long tone musculature. I often do my yoga first thing out of bed. Yoga is a great wake up and easy to do in your room with a DVD, Netflix, or Youtube.

- Men, Yes you still have time. Once you begin exercising, your man hormones will kick in and your body will transform. Be progressive, but build into it slowly so you don't injure yourself and quit. Quitting will get you nowhere!

- No, you won't see immediate results on the scale. Muscle weighs more than fat so you will probably see the scale go up before it goes down. Stay consistent and give it time.

Hi5 Action Steps

What to choose
- Begin with walking regularly to get your mind and body acquainted with the idea of exercising.

- When you are ready, incorporate interval training exercises. You can begin with 5 minutes of a small routine (ie: lunges, pushups, air squats) after your walk and progress from there.

- Choose from the list of exercises from the back of the book to create your routine.

- Find an area that you designate for your exercising. It doesn't have to be big. Over the years I have exercised in my bedroom, the living room, the kitchen, the garage and even the bathroom. The bathroom was my favorite because I could lock everyone out!

- Learn how to do the exercises properly by visiting www.hi5health-network.com or Google or youtube.

- Post the exercise you choose on the wall so it is there when you need it.

- Keep the tools that you need easily available.

- Set an appointment with yourself and keep it. Keep your appointment even if you just do stretching or deep breathing. **Commitment begins with showing up!**

Sometimes I only have 5 minutes or no minutes to exercise but I often go out to the area that I exercise just to show up and stay in the routine which keeps me on track. It is so important to commit to exercise 5 days per week because if you miss one, it just becomes one of your free days. If you don't use it as a free day, then you'll have no guilt because you exercised 4 days, which is really great. From personal experience, if you try to schedule 3 times per week for longer periods of time, something will always come up to mess up your schedule.

In the cave man days, exercise was done everyday anyway, so five days is really a break for us.

Menu of exercises:

This is not a big deal, just choose a few that you can do, make a list, learn how to do them correctly, and post them up where you can see them when it is time to exercise. Mix up your routine to include core exercises, lower body and upper body exercise.

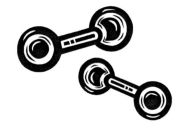

Triple Threat:

When I was a young momma with 4 small children, growing our business, and trying to be super mom, my husband, myself, a few nephews and my sister-in-law began the Triple Threat. The Triple Threat saved me!

Five days per week, on our own, we had to do 100 push-ups, 50 lunges on each leg, and 100 abdominal exercises. We became accountable to each other and we stayed active even though we had no time. My nephews had more time than I did but this gave them the kick start they needed.

- 100 Push-ups- I did the girl push-ups. If this is difficult, then just alternate with holding a plank position for a period of time.

- 100 Abs - We just did basic crunches, but now there are so many other options. www.hi5healthnetwork.com

- 50/50 Lunges - This was the best. Sometimes I would crawl out of bed half asleep and start doing my lunges and that would wake me up. Learn how to use proper form www.hi5healthnetwork.com or Youtube.

Ab Pulsing Exercises

Another sister-in-law who is a professional dancer taught me how to do Ab Pulsing exercises. These exercises can be done anywhere and everywhere.

While sitting or standing, concentrate on pulling your belly button in toward your spine. Don't raise your shoulders or hold your breath. Once you have pulled your belly button in, make very small pulsing contractions to work the core muscle. You should be able to talk while doing these abdominal exercises.

At the time I was traveling weekly and I made it a game to see how many contractions I could do till I got to my destination. That is the summer I had my best abs.

Commuters and travelers make it happen!

Tools to use:

- Interval timer
- Timer
- Music

Optional tools to use:

- dumbbells
- punching bag and gloves
- weighted balls or med balls
- Bands
- Physio ball
- Yokebar (see www.yokebar.com)
- Rebounder
- Jump rope
- and your body!!

Visit www.hi5healthsystem.com for resources of tools and exercises.

Hi5 Action Steps:

- **Pull out your calendar and schedule your daily 10-25 minute exercise appointments.**
- **Make a list of things you would enjoy doing.**

- Gather the exercise equipment you need and keep ready at all times.

- Show up to your appointment everyday even for 5 minutes.

- Find an exercise buddy. This is the best way to stay committed, but don't use it as an excuse to not exercise if your buddy is a flake.

When will you exercise each day?

_____

_____

_____

What exercises will you include in your routine?

_____

_____

_____

Who can be an exercise partner or help you stay accountable?

_____

_____

_____

What is _your_ "why" to exercise?

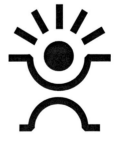

1. Eat whatever you want.
2. Get-away and relieve stress.
3. Keep weight off.
4. Look tone and fit.
5. Feel sexy.
6. Live a long life.
7. Slow down the visual signs of aging.
8. Prevent heart disease or some other serious disease.
9. Socially interact more comfortably.

10. Feel good and feel alive.
11. Do the right thing.
12. All of the above

What is your "why"? I can honestly say my reasons are all of the above. It took me a long time to say I really enjoy exercising, but I think it has more to do with my attitude change.

_____
_____
_____
_____
_____

Straight talk with Denise

Hands down, exercise is the best thing that you can do to slow down the aging process, detox the body, lose weight, have more energy, lower depression, and improve virtually every aspect of your health. If you did nothing else but exercise, you would be on the right track. Trust me I have tried everything else. I have searched all the short cuts. We must move our bodies DAILY! But on the bright side everything counts. Walking at the mall, cleaning house, gardening, dancing and playing with the kids all count. So have fun and get healthy in the process.

Chapter 5:
Fun is an attitude

- *The flavor that makes it all happen*
- *The secret sauce of life*

What soap is to the body, laughter is to the soul.
unknown author

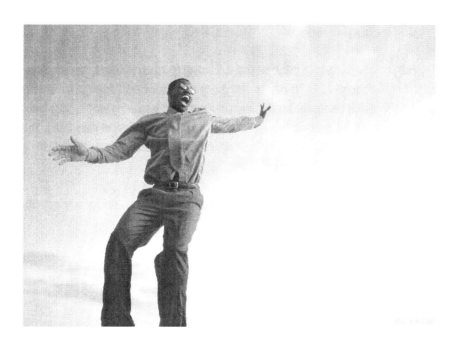

Fun is an attitude

Why?
If you did nothing else in this book but incorporate an attitude of fun and laughter, you would instantly strengthen your heart, boosts your immune system, have more energy and yes even lose weight. Can you believe it's the most effective way to improve our health and life and is often times the hardest to do?

Fun is an attitude we choose to adopt. It isn't just the things we do on vacation. Fun is how we find life exciting and people interesting. Imagine the worst possible scenario in your life for a moment. Now look at your current life. It may not be perfect but it is pretty darn good if you are breathing and you have people to love and things to learn.

Wikipedia definition:

Fun is the enjoyment of pleasure and, according to Johan Huizinga, "an absolutely primary category of life, familiar to everybody at a glance right down to the animal level."[1] Fun may be encountered in many human activities during work, social functions, recreation and play, and even seemingly mundane activities of daily living. The distinction between enjoyment and fun is difficult to articulate but real,[2] fun being a more spontaneous, playful, and active event.

The perception of time is shortened when one is "having fun".[3]

Fun is often described as *doing what you enjoy*, which can be any activity imaginable

Humans are a funny thing in that we all desire to be happy, but it seems like we move away from the things that actually bring us joy. Adopting an attitude of fun will certainly bring more joy to your life.

Having fun boosts your energy. My kids always seem to be tired when it is time to clean house, but tell them we are going to Disneyland after we clean and they have enough energy to clean 10 houses.

Humor

Laugh more, it's like a drug!! Laughter is the physiological response to an attitude in our mind in response to something in our environment or our thoughts. When we laugh the muscles of the body contract and relax similar to healing relaxation type of techniques. The stress hormone cortisol decreases and endorphins are released similar to exercise! The breathing pattern changes in a way that increases oxygen and releases toxins.

Laughing takes the attention off your situation and yourself and helps you gain a new perspective. In his book, Anatomy of an Illness, Norman Cousins explains how he overcame a rare and painful disease using laugh therapy.

Best of all, laughing is contagious so hang out with people with a sense of humor and you will live younger and be healthier. The opposite is also true; hang out with downers and you will be down. Limit your time around negative people if you are serious about losing weight, boosting your immune system, and living an all around healthy life. If you happen to be married to a grumpy negative person, wear a permanent smile and create an environment in your home that is difficult to be grumpy in.

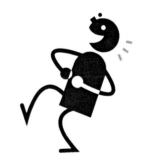

Live Alive

Open your eyes to the life around you. Too many people are zooming around doing their daily activities with a melancholy dryness. The loss of zest for life creeps up from pressures, responsibilities, disappointments, and set-backs. You are not alone. In my 20's I thought I could do anything, in my 30's I realized I could do nothing, and now in my 40's I woke up to understand who I am and not worry about what I can or can't do but to enjoy each moment and live alive. Don't wait until you're in your 40's! If you're in your 40's carpe diem! If you are past your 40's waste no more time dwelling on the past and take charge of your greatness and live with purpose.

Trick Yourself (again)

If the whole idea of adopting a fun attitude doesn't come naturally, simply trick yourself. Tell yourself that you are a fun person, life is exciting and people are interesting. Get a few books to keep around that you know will make you smile such as book of quotes, motivational books, comical books, or funny pictures. Find movies that make you laugh and watch them frequently. Visit comedy clubs.

SMILE!! Best way to trick yourself is to smile. Try it. It is really hard to be grumpy when you are smiling.

Tell the people around you that you are working on being more positive for your health's sake and see if they would help you. I had a friend who frequently spoke negative comments consciously, or unconsciously, I am not sure. I finally had to tell her that her negative talk had to stop because either my positive was going to affect her or her negative was going to affect me and if that happens I am going to be mad. She laughed because I said it with a light heart, but she made a conscious effort to use positive words around me. I am happy to say she is now an optimistic person and the best side affect has been her improved relationship with her children.

Schedule it

Simple enough right? Get your calendar out and plan movie night, comedy night, go to bookstores and hunt for the comedy section, schedule play time with children, or walks with your spouse. Find that positive person in your life and spend time in their presence. Schedule it on your Hi5 Health Grid.

In Your Mind

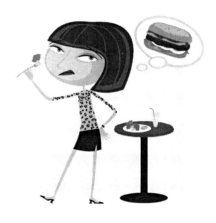

Do you find yourself in a perpetual conversation of 'if only....'? If only my kids weren't so messy. If only my husband made more money. If only I lost weight.

If only I was healthier. If only I had a house, a nicer car, more friends, better family, better kids, better spouse, ... STOP! It's all in your mind. The Hi5 Mindset is about the conversation you are having in your head.

Control your thoughts, control your attitude.
Control your attitude, control your choices.
Control your choices, control your life.

Mama T & Auntie Claire Factor

Do you know anyone that has such a fun attitude that they can make a trip to the DMV a bowl of laughs? Maybe that's you!! I do hope so, then you would be leaps ahead toward a better health. If you do know someone who lives life with a fun attitude, hang around and let it rub off on you and bring that attitude back to other parts of your life.

I have two sister-in-laws who can laugh while stuck in traffic or standing in line at the grocery store. Auntie Claire and Mama T have their fair share of nonsense in life, but they make a conscious effort to do the things to ease the load of stresses in life.

Mama T's tool box of fun:

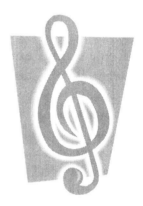

- Music, music and anything about music!

- She loves to listen to live music, whether professionals or amateur

- She chooses to be around children

- Plays with her Bulldog

- Never watches the news

- Favorite word is "whatever!"

- She makes up silly songs and twist words around that make you laugh

- Goes to church

- She is totally devoted to her family and loves them as they are

- Mama T visits Disneyland every year

- Makes time to hang out at Starbucks and laugh

Auntie Claire's tool box of fun:

- She recites these mantras whenever she gets down: 'Only your own thoughts create your own pain', 'I completely and deeply love and accept myself', 'Everything is done for you not to you.'

Fun is an attitude

- Claire often taps the top of her head, under her eyes and around her temples while reciting these mantras. Silly?? yes! It is so silly and so effective and it makes you laugh.

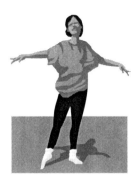

- She uses magnet necklaces to keep her energy balanced

- Claire gardens and takes regular walks

- She dances anytime as her heart moves her

- Loves life and people

- Claire finds silly in the mundane day to day

- Starbucks hang out time to laugh is a must

The most amazing thing is how many lives they affect and they don't even realize it. I have been with them around town where people come up to say hello as if they have been family friends forever only to find out they just met the person from the last time they visited this particular store or restaurant. Mama T and Auntie Claire make strangers feel like they are friends of the family.

Hi5 Action Steps:

- List things that you enjoy doing and seeing on your Hi5 Health Grid so you don't forget when things get busy.

- SMILE

- LAUGH

What things do you like to do that are fun?

_____

_____

Do you smile and laugh enough?

_____

_____

_____

What makes you smile?

_____

_____

_____

Who can you hang around with that makes you laugh?

_____

_____

_____

Straight Talk with Denise

Life is short, live in the moment.

Chapter 6:
Family and Friends

How do you rally the Troops?

"Only a life lived for others is a life worth while."
Albert Einstein

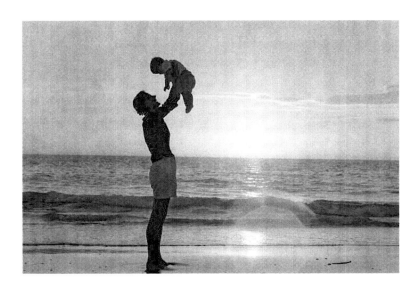

Family/ Friends

Family and friends are your resource, your tool, your why, the flame that keeps you motivated, the wind beneath your wings. Sound poetic? Or are you dealing with an unsupportive spouse, unappreciative kids and cynical friends? Either way, let's look at ways to harness the power in the community of family and friends to keep you on track.

Your Why

What makes you get up in the morning and go to work? What makes you brush your teeth, dress nice, smell nice, and wash your face? Don't answer, "I just want to feel good about myself". In reality we do those things so that we are pleasant and appealing to the people we interact in our circle of socialization. When was the last time you woke up with goop in your eyes, hair array, still in your PJs and got in the car and headed to the grocery store? We actually clean up because we care about how we influence others.

What greater influence our family has on us and we on them. So use it consciously to accomplish awesome things like creating a healthy home and body.

Let your family and friends become your drive, your support, and your resource.

How do we rally the troops?

1. Tell them that you need their help to keep you on track and motivated.

2. Ask them to be understanding and patient as you adjust to trying new foods and a new exercise schedule.

3. Explain to them that it is going to be
a big adventure as you discover new
things about how the body works.

4. Post your Hi5 Health System Grid
in places where everyone can see it
so they can be familiar with what
you are doing.

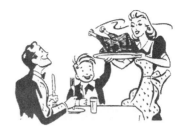

5. Ask them not to give ANY negative comments whether you follow the system or not. Because you are not trying to be perfect,
you are just trying to move toward a healthier direction.

6. Make a Motivation poster with words, phrases and pictures that get
you excited about what an energetic healthy life will offer and post
it where the family can see. Make sure you have a picture of them
on it so they know they are a valuable part of your journey.

How do you not suffocate them with your ideas?

1. Be strong on your path but be patient and not surprised when they
don't jump on board.

2. Make it fun and not forceful.

3. Create a healthy environment for them to live in. Open the win-
dows, de-clutter the house, make fresh fruit available on the table,
and put music on that creates a happy atmosphere.

4. Wear a smile!

5. Give them grace; they are not where you are. Who knows if they
will ever get there, but they will absolutely be influenced if you
keep it a fun and a positive experience.

6. Oh yeah, most important, don't remove all the junk food in your
home at once or you will start a war.

Seasons of Life

Remember this: Life happens in seasons. So roll with it! When my children were small, I exercised in the bathroom before getting in the shower because I knew once the day started it was non-stop and I wouldn't have time. As the seasons changed, we adjusted. My meals are healthier when I plan ahead, but I often get off track with busyness. No big deal, just get back on track again.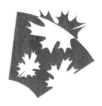

Smile

A smile can change and soothe the worst circumstances. A smile can change your mood and attitude in a snap. Try being grumpy and angry while smiling non-stop.

Love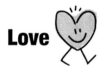

Tell them that you love them frequently even when you don't feel it. It may sound too simple, but it is the life blood of our existence. Without feeling and knowing that we are loved daily we lose our passion.

Time schedule

It's simple, if you don't schedule quality time devoted to your family, they will consciously or subconsciously sabotage your best efforts.

Tell them

The greatest thing you can do to become a person of influence is tell people how valuable they are. People everywhere are starving for affirmation and attention. Make people around you flourish simply by your words. You wouldn't let your child starve for a week without food. Don't let a day go by without telling the people you care about how important they are. For humans, the need to be valued is so strong that some people will spend their whole life trying to fill that emptiness with food, negativism, bad relationships and other destructive behaviors. Determine to uplift the people in your circle of network and watch how it lifts you up in the process.

Hi5 Action Steps

- List the people that are important to you on your Hi5 Health Grid.

- Tell them every day that they are valuable.

- Think of something special to do each week with the people you love.

- Create an Inspirational Poster to remind you of the wonderful people and things that you love in life. Include words and pictures that inspire you. Post it somewhere you will see frequently.

Who are the people that need your love and attention?

_____

_____

_____

_____

Do they genuinely know how important they are? Do you tell them frequently?

_____

_____

What things can you do to get away from the demands of day to day to just focus on the people important to you?

_____

_____

_____

_____

Straight talk with Denise

Rallying the troops is harder than it sounds, but don't give up, you won't have regrets. Look around as you go about your day and see people rushing about in their zone. You have no idea the challenges they deal with, so make a point to be friendly and kind. Say "Hello" and smile because it just might be the only affirmation they get.

Chapter 7:
Faith

What you believe is how you think
How you think is how you act
How you act is who you become

Warning!!
It takes more than just believing to be healthy. Faith might give you comfort and peace, but it won't take the french fries off your hips. Take responsibility and look at all the pieces together.

Faith is the art of holding on to things your reason has once ac-
cepted in spite of your changing mood
CS Lewis

One life is all we have and we live it as we believe in living it. But
to sacrifice what you are and to live without belief, that is a fate
more terrible than dying.
Joan of Arc

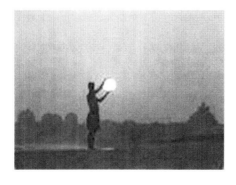

Faith

Shortest chapter in the book, but toughest to write! Since it is such a sensitive topic I pondered on whether I should eliminate it all together. If I did, this whole book wouldn't work or make sense. Your faith is what you believe and what you believe is how you think and how you think is what you act upon. You are going to believe in something and it is up to you to discover what it will be. Most importantly, it is your faith that gives you hope and purpose.

We are all being mentally programmed, so find good things to believe in. Remember our goal here is to create a health foundation that is strong and functions with purpose, so discover what drives you. What moves you and harness that!

Faith is the confident belief or trust in the truth or trustworthiness of a person, concept or thing.[1][2] The English word is thought to date from 1200–50, from the Latin *fidem* or *fidēs*, meaning trust, derived from the verb *fīdere*, to trust.[1]

Why is faith important to my health?

- Foundation of faith is love. When you love others unselfishly, good things start flooding your way including chemicals in your body that boosts your immune system.

- Having faith that your life has meaning will absolutely give you the drive to keep going. This is where passion comes from.

- Faith is a knowing that you are not fighting this life alone.

- Peace is a great benefit to living in faith. Peace in your spirit will decrease your stress and depression better than any drug.

- Faith gives you hope in the goodness in people even when they are not showing it.

How?

- Pray and start asking the questions.

- Have an attitude of gratitude. When you don't feel very grateful, remind yourself that there is always someone in worse circumstances than you, then smile and watch the feelings change.

- Reprogram your brain with words that build you up and not tear you down. The conversation you have in your head has the most impact to your outcome in everything.

- Eliminate guilt! Look at everything as a learning experience and let go of the guilt.

- Use affirmations. It may sound crazy but it works! My favorite is "I can do this. I am great. I love life and people are beautiful".

- Your faith should build you up. If the faith you're following doesn't make you a better person, find a different one.

- Give. Give of your time and resources to help others unselfishly during this 5 weeks and see how it impacts you.

- Find a group of people who share your beliefs and gather frequently to learn from each other. Word of caution, those people are growing in their faith too so don't expect perfection.

Hi5 Action Steps:

1. Explore your beliefs

2. Beware of negative self-talk; it will always sabotage your efforts. Post positive affirmations where you can see them frequently.

3. List a few things you can do each week for the 5 weeks that helps you explore and grow your faith. Add those to your Hi5 Health Grid.

What is your faith based on?

_____

_____

_____

_____

What can you do daily to strengthen your faith?

_____

_____

What is your purpose in this world?

_____

_____

_____

_____

Straight talk with Denise

My faith gives me peace and hope that I couldn't imagine living without. Everything seems to make sense and when it doesn't my faith reassures me that I am not doing this life aimlessly and alone. I have had countless doubtful moments and it is those times that I ask God lots of questions. My questions are honest and my spirit is wanting to understand. Then as crazy as it seems, answers begin to reveal themselves to me in journaling, in books, in people, in movies, in song, my senses and then I know.

Your life has meaning and value. You can make a difference when you live with purpose. Whatever your purpose is in life-better health brings you along that journey with more energy and effectiveness.

Chapter 8:
Making it Last

It was character that got us out of bed, commitment that moved us into action, and discipline that enabled us to follow through.
~ Zig Ziglar

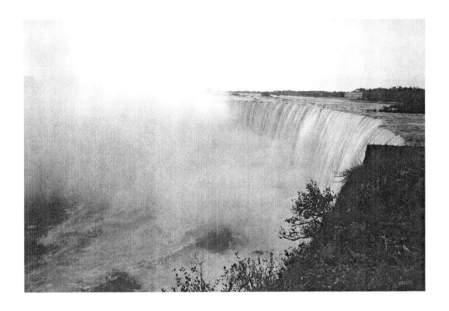

Making it Last

Making all the wonderful health habits last can be difficult because our bodies will always try to go back to the familiar. The body always tries to go back to its equilibrium which is all of our old habits. How do you make it last?

Journey

Like a road trip across country. So excited and energetic when you begin then fatigue, pit stops, detours, and change in weather alters the trip a bit. But you don't give up you just keep going! On this health journey you can take the long way, the ugly way, the bumpy way, and who knows if you will even make it. Take the new paved freeway in a nice car and you will get there feeling good.

Eb and Flow

Nothing in this life is static. We get all stressed when there is change, but it is the one thing we know for sure - everything will change. If you have children you know the dynamics will change frequently so roll with it. Create healthy habits that are so easy and 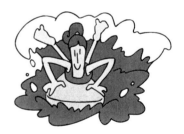 second nature that as life ebs and flows, it doesn't throw you off. It is only your health foundation that will determine how you cope and adjust with life's ups and downs.

No Stop and Start

Whether you think you are going to start living healthy or not doesn't really matter because you already are living in some health manner. Your health doesn't start or stop, it just keeps going as time passes, we call it aging. My goal for this book was to give you the tools to help you age in the simplest way and with class. Make the first positive health choices today and you will reap exponential benefit tomorrow.

2 Ways to Create Change

ONLY two ways to create change. ALERT!! This is the most important piece of this chapter. There are only two ways to create change!!

Ready to know how??

*   Heightened emotional experience and spaced repetition.

Heightened emotional experience is something traumatic like a diagnosis of cancer or other serious disease. A family death or divorce could catapult one into change. Although very effective, don't wait for that!

A better way to make this healthy lifestyle last is with spaced repetition. Have you ever heard 'out of sight, out of mind'? That phrase is the same concept. When something is fresh in your mind it is easier to keep up, but as soon as you spend less time thinking about it, the actions will fade away. This isn't about lack of self discipline or commitment; it is about 'out of sight out of mind'.

This is when guilt creeps in. We all hate guilt so we do whatever it takes to avoid it. This includes the healthy habits which caused the guilt in the first place. Finally, we convince ourselves it doesn't matter anyway.

Spaced repetition is key, which is why you need to keep this book and others around you at all times! I want to give you charts and wallet reminders to keep the Hi5 Health System fresh in your mind. Everyday will have its own challenges that will try to trip you up on this journey, but spaced repetition will keep you on track. Visit Hi5 Health Network online community, it was created for you. It's a great opportunity to discover what other people are doing on their health journey and learn new things. Explore the website, create your own profile and tell us how your journey is progressing.

Tools for Spaced Repetition:

Hi5 Health System Grid posted where you will see it frequently (refrigerator, bathroom mirror, bedroom, closet door, in car, at work etc.)

- Online health newsletters

- Online health community www.hi5healthnetwork.com

- Inspiration Poster of people you love, things you love, words and images that inspire you.

- Accountability or workout partner

- Personal trainer or lifestyle coach

Mind Reprogram

Something is programming your mind at all times. It's nothing to be afraid of or avoid. Those that understand this reality harness the tools needed to program their thoughts exactly the way they want. Remember your thoughts, determine your actions, and your actions determine your outcome. Sound easy? Not really, but simply by understanding how powerful your mind is will make you stronger.

+ mindset = + life
- mindset = - life

Sleep

The fastest way to derail EVERYTHING is lack of sleep. The effects on your health are even worse than stress or smoking! If it is impossible to get 7-8 hrs of sleep per night, squeeze a nap in to put you back on track. Power naps of even 10 minutes have great effect on your health. If you have trouble taking a nap, simply lying down to rest and closing your eyes will provide great benefit.

Attitude:

You will have disappointing days when it seems like none of this health stuff works. You still feel yucky and overweight and that is when the negative attitude sets in and we tend to give up. Negative self talk and give up attitude perpetuates and it's over! That is when you dig down deep and laugh! Do whatever it takes to change your attitude.

Time

You have TIME. If you think you do not have time, imagine how much time you would have if you suddenly broke your leg or got really sick. Ok, let's stay positive. Imagine how much time you would have if you were offered a million dollar shopping spree or a free trip around the world. Suddenly we have time if the motivation is great enough.

Why wait for the perfect time. Start NOW! Pull out your calendar and determine when you can fit in 25 minutes to exercise. Write it down on your calendar. Hopefully, your exercise will become like a favorite TV show. Most of us will drop what we are doing to not miss our show. Trust me, 25 minutes of exercise everyday will make you happier.

If you are like me, you need things automated; print your Hi5 Health System Grid and post them at several places around the house. Post affirmations around the house to help with spaced repetition. Visit www.hi5healthnetwork to download your free Hi5 Health Grid and affirmations. Plan your meals and write it down so you do not have to think about what to eat when you are in hungry mode. This may seem like it takes a lot of time to plan frequently, but eventually it will become second nature and then a lifestyle.

Resources

- Get your resources available and easy to use so you have no excuses.

- Make a shelf for your supplements.

- Keep your Hi5 Health Grid posted where you can see it daily.

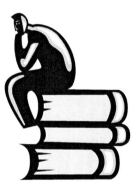

- Make healthy snacks available at all times.

- Plan your meals

- Have your list of exercises that you like posted on a wall where you can see.

- Have your music and timers available for exercise time.

- Prepare to combat negative self talk and lack of motivation. Make a list of ideas on your Hi5 Heath Grid. My list includes: watch a funny movie, go to the beach, go for a walk, journal write, read my affirmations, eat fruit or smile.

Keep thinking of ways to automate that work into your unique routine.

Photo Diary

For the 5 weeks of the Hi5 Health System you will take photos of everything you eat. Awareness is key for creating new habits. By gathering photos of what you eat over time you will notice patterns in how you make good choices and bad choices.

Shopping

The art shopping! Ugh I wish there was an easy step by step that really really worked. The truth is you still have to plan and do it. There are some great shopping guides like the one from Bill Phillips in Body for Life.

The simplest way is to plan the dinner meals on the Hi5 Health Grid based on the protein for each dinner followed by big veggie/ salad selection for that meal.

Make one or two meals habitual, like oatmeal or egg for breakfast and salad or 1/2 sandwich for lunch. Eliminate the stress of trying to decide what to eat by rotating your favorite options. When we shop during hungry or hurried times without a plan, we will definitely deviate from our health goals.

Straight talk with Denise

I know this is not as easy as reading a book and everything falls into place. It will be a daily conscious effort. An effort that often seems not worth it. It is easy to think that none of these choices matter. It is like a drip of water under the kitchen sink. One drip is not a big deal but over time the constant drip can create so much damage. That is like the daily choices we make. Skipping a few days of not exercising not a big deal but over time, so much damage. Similarly, one diet soda is not a big deal but over time the damage of artificial sweetener can have catastrophic effects.

Trust me, the effort is worth it on so many levels. Once you complete the 5 weeks, you can decide to do it again. Evaluate, make any adjustments and do it again and again until these new lifestyle habits are part of your daily routine. It will become second nature and less and less of an effort.

Chapter 9:
Beyond Foundation

"The Journey is the Reward"
Chinese Proverb

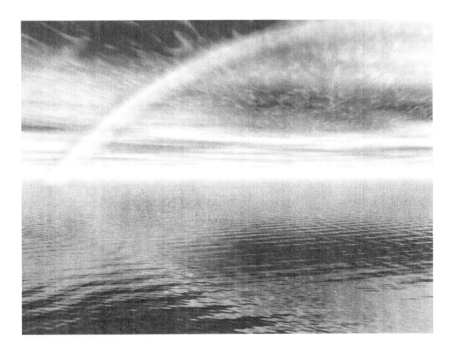

Beyond Foundation

Moving beyond foundation on your health journey can include:

- Complimentary therapies: acupuncture, chiropractic, colonics, massage, hypnotherapy, homeopathy, fasting, counseling etc.

- New goal specific diet plans

- Herbs or unique supplements

- Personal trainer

- Natural Hormone therapy

- Detox/ Cleansing programs

Since everything is based on a strong healthy foundation, you will be amazed at how many of your common ailments will fix themselves using the Hi5 Health System. However, many of the serious or long standing health challenges will require therapies beyond foundation.

Often times, it was that big health challenge that motivated us to make changes in our lifestyle in the first place. By building your health foundation first, your body and mind will be ready and prepared for whatever therapy or advanced program you choose.

The Mind is half the battle

If you have no ailments, congrats. Savor what you have and get aggressive building your foundation. If you or a loved one does have an ailment to work on, be more aggressive at building a foundation, and research other natural therapies. Most importantly, celebrate that which is great about your health and be confident that there is something out there just for you.

Half of the physical battle is your mind keeping you from healing. Look into laugh therapy or spiritual therapy or, my favorite, go to the ocean. Take the mind aspect very seriously when trying to heal. A negative mindset and stress will not allow your body to heal itself.

Healing Crisis

No matter what healing path you choose beyond foundation, sometimes the body feels worse before it feels better. That is called a healing crisis. This can be very difficult because you could get more sick or very tired as the body tries to purge or heal. You can adjust your program, but don't give up. Remember, your body didn't get to this state overnight and it will not fix itself overnight.

Words of Encouragement for Crisis state

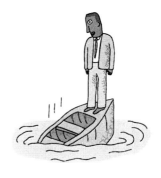

It goes without saying that everyone is unique and this is by no means a one size fits all. It is however, a framework to build your foundation. The pieces to the Hi5 Health System are fundamental key ingredients to life. Use it as a springboard to accomplish even greater goals than imagined.

I am not a doctor and this is not a prescription, only words of encouragement and a roadmap to follow. I know what it is like when you want to be well or you want to help your loved ones get well, but you don't know where to start. Because the body is amazing at healing itself, I still recommend starting at the foundation. The difference while in crisis would be to inquire outside help or other therapies in conjunction with building your foundation.

If you are serious about healing, be determined and know that your body wants to be healthy and pain free. Know that there is something out there that can help you reach your optimal health. Sometimes you heal just by being aggressive with building a healthy foundation and sometimes you need more.

Never give up. A crisis is an opportunity to see what your body can do.

My third child had severe eczema as a baby that put me on a mission to help her heal. It was so severe that if her skin was exposed to air she would scratch and make it bleed. My husband put a large butcher paper on the wall and we wrote down suggestions and ideas from books, internet or other people. We tried everything from oatmeal bathes to chiropractic. I was even told to dunk her in the Red Sea. I am glad I didn't have to go that far.

I read several books and finally found one that really resonated. I told my husband that I was taking her to see the author of the book. I told no one at the time because I didn't want any negative energy. My attitude was whether it worked or not I was going to try. It worked! Dr Andrew Kail from Phoenix Arizona used a desensitizing technique in combination with enzyme therapy. The two factors to her success were her strong foundation and our "whatever it takes" attitude.

Final Note from Denise

As I take a deep breath in finishing this book for you, I ask myself what else can I give you. What else can I offer that will make this pursuit of health simple? I wish I could hang out with you, shop with you, exercise with you and sit around and enjoy a cup of tea and talk about great things. I would love to hear about your family, your hobbies, your vacations, and your dreams. Because I bet you are amazing! I bet you are interesting. Until then, know that I am cheering for you and wish you all the best that this life has to offer.

I believe with all my heart that if you work on creating a strong healthy foundation, life will bring you abundance in every way possible and you truly will have it all.

What now?
Get started!

Visit our online community to learn and be inspired. Spaced repetition is your only way toward changing your mindset and creating a healthy lifestyle. So, keep reading, learning and exploring. Send me an email and let me know what you have discovered. If you find a great restaurant or healthy recipe share it with us. If you find something new and simple that has improved your health, tells us about it.

www.hi5healthnetwork.com

Chapter 10:
Resources

Note: The list below are some of my favorite books that have guided and inspired me on my health journey. Many of the authors listed have several books that I recommend you examine. You can find a more extensive list on our website www.hi5healthnetwork.com. Visit your local bookstore or library and begin exploring and creating your own health library. Many libraries sell used and donated books for almost nothing

Books:

Tony O'Donnell C.N.C Naturopath, Miracle Red Super Foods that Heal

Elson Haas, M.D. , Stay Healthy with the Seasons

Jordan S. Rubin, The Makers Diet for Weight Loss

Bill Phillips, Eating for Life

Charlotte Gerson, The Gerson Therapy

Michael F. Roizen, M.D. & Mehmet C. Oz, M.D., Staying Young-The Owner's Manual for Extending your Warranty

Helice "Sparky" Bridges, Who I am Makes a Difference

Patricia Bragg, Bragg Healthy Lifestyle

Donna Gates, The Body Ecology Diet

Konrad Kail, N.D. & Bobbi Laurence with Burton Goldberg, Allergy Free

Felicia Drury Kliment, The Acid Alkaline Balance Diet

Melina B. Jampolis, M.D. , The No Time to Lose Diet

Jeff Victoroff, M.D. Saving Your Brain

Tim Ferris, The Four Hour Work-Week

Norman Vincent Peale, Enthusiasm Makes the Difference

Florence Scovel Shinn, The Wisdom of Florence Scovel Shinn

John R. Lee, M.D. What your Doctor May Not Tell You About Breast Cancer.

Dr. Michael Colgan, Sports Nutrition Guide

Kevin Trudeau, Natural Cures "They" Don't Want You to Know About

Judith J. Wurtman, Ph.D., Managing Your Mind and Mood Through Food

Michael Van Straten, Healing Foods

Michael A. Schmidt, Lendon H. Smith and Keith W. Sehnert, Beyond Antibiotics

Kriss Carr, Crazy Sexy Cancer Tips

Andrew Weil, M.D., Reader's Digests Guide to Natural Medicine

Canyon Ranch, Great Tastes

Gail E. Dennison, Paul E. Dennison, Ph.D and Jerry V. Teplitz, J.D., Ph.D, Brain Gym

David Hoffman, The Herbal Handbook

Joseph Pizzorno, N.D. Total Wellness

Janet Zand, LAe, OMD, Rachel Walton, RN and Bob Rountree, M.D., Smart Medicine for a Healthier Child

Burton Goldenberg Group, Alternative Medicine

Julia Careon, The Artist's Way

Nicholas Perricone, M.D., Dr Perricone 7 Secrets to Beauty, Health and Longevity

Jon Gordon, Energy Addict 101

Frank Lipman, M.D. Total Renewal

Christine Northrup, M.D. Women's Bodies Women's Wisdom

Websites:
www.hi5healthnetwork.com
Online community for like minded "hey, we want to get healthy" people.
Downloads Hi5 Health Grid, daily tracker, videos, chats, and so much more!

Popular websites that have great information
www.droz.com
www.drmercola.com
www.bodyecologydiet.com

GLYCEMIC FOODS TO CHOOSE

These are great options when choosing carbohydrates because they cause the sugar to enter the cells at a slower steady pace as compared to table sugar, processed foods, fruit juices, sweets, candy, soft drinks, white rice, white bread and white pastas.

<u>Choose</u>
ALL VEGETABLES
barley beans, brown rice, couscous, lentils, oatmeal, potato, quinoa, rye, squash

whole wheat multigrain bread, corn, high fiber unsweetened cereal, whole wheat pasta, whole wheat tortilla

almond butter, almonds, avocados, coconut oil, olive oil, flaxseed, peanut butter, pumpkin seeds, nuts, plain yogurt

*Foods that are highly debatable are potatoes, brown rice, and whole wheat. Simply eat these foods in moderation and pay close attention to how your body responds. Try a short fast from these foods then slowly re-enter them into your diet and make note of how you feel.

*Glycemic Index does not necessarily indicate the nutritional value of the food only how it affects the insulin level in the body. For example, foods sweetened with artificial sweeteners will be listed as low glycemic, but are extremely unhealthy and should not be part of anyone's meal plan who wants to lose weight or be healthy.

Note: The Glycemic Index is only for carbohydrates therefore, you will not see for example chicken, beef, pork, fish, turkey, eggs, or cheese. When choosing a protein choose lean and natural (free from antibiotics and hormones) whenever possible. Include a protein portion at each meal for steady sustained energy and controlled appetite.

"MUST HAVE" FOOD STAPLE LIST

- FRUIT!!
- VARIETY OF VEGETABLES
- Lean meats
- Eggs
- Oatmeal
- Almonds
- Beans (fresh and canned)
- High fiber and high protein cereal
- Variety of fruits
- Tuna in water
- Yogurt
- Kephur
- Sauerkraut &/or Kimchee
- Brown rice

Whole wheat tortillas
Whole wheat pasta
Hummus
Garlic
Frozen meats no sauce
Frozen vegetables no sauce
Lemons
Olive oil
Limes
Cottage cheese
Variety seasonings
Whole wheat bread

- High nutrient rich specialty drinks (protein shakes, fiber drinks, green drinks, super fruits, coconut water, carrot juice, wheat grass etc.)

Remember: When planning your meals include a protein, fat and carbohydrate at each meal. Think wholesome foods that come as natural as possible. The more processed the food the harder it is for your body to utilize it for fuel and it becomes dangerous instead of helpful. Because you will be eating 5 meals per day you can easily cut your portion sizes in half and still feel completely satisfied. In addition, once you feed your body the nutrients it needs from the supplements, your cells won't be starving therefore, you will lose the need to overeat.

Also, if you find yourself hungry between meals, drink a glass of water, take a walk or snack on carrots or some other vegetable.

EXERCISES FOR INTERVAL TRAINING

Here is a list of exercise to choose, to make your interval training. Safety is priority! Ask a fitness professional to teach you how to do the exercises that you choose or visit www.hi5healthnetwork.com or youtube for great demonstrations.

Optional ways to design your routine

- You can do a few exercises in a cycle then repeat the cycle till you reach your designated time.

- Choose a small number of exercises and repeat the cycle or choose several to do an intense workout.

- Whether you are starting with 10 minutes after your walk or a 25 minute routine, mix up your routine with a few lower body, upper body, abdominals and cardio exercise.

Don't overwhelm yourself with too many exercises. Too much thinking diminishes the intensity of a great workout.

The exercise menu below can be done without equipment. So anyone can make up an interval routine anywhere! If you have equipment, simply incorporate them and you will add variety to your routine.

Lower body

- Forward Lunge

- Reverse Lunge

- Side lunge

- Jump Lunge

- Lunge followed by raise back leg

- Reverse lunge followed by knee raise

- Walking lunge

- Air Squats

- Jump air squats

- Ice skaters

- Burpees

- Calf raises

- Mountain climber

Upper body

- Plank - straight back, no sagging of the hips, pull belly button in to contract abdominals

- Push up - Perfect form is vital so be sure to research examples.

  Lots of variation *Incline to make easier ie bench or wall *Decline push up for very advanced *Balance feet or hands on ball *Knee position (aka girl push ups *Military push up * Diamond push up

- Tricep dip (use a stable step such as a chair, bleacher, bench or box)

Cardio (these are great in between exercise)

- Jumping jacks

- Run in place with high knees

- Dance

- Jump rope

- Shadow boxing

Abdominal exercise

- Basic abdominal crunch

- Reverse abdominal crunch

- Oblique crunch

- Abdominal bicycles

- Abdominal pulsing

- Abdominal seated leg lift

- Salsa or belly dancing exercise for abdominals

Triple Threat (simplest routine that saved me in my busiest times of life)

Focus on keeping abdominals contracted throughout lunges and push ups.

- 50/50 Lunges - Great for strengthening the large fat burning muscle groups.

- 50 push ups - If you maintain belly button pulled in this becomes a great full body workout.

- 100 abdominal exercises (any variety)

Optional Equipment for Exercise

- Punching bag and gloves

- Physio ball

- Weighted medicine balls

- Dumbbells

- Kettlebells

- Resistance bands

- Barbell

- Jump rope

- Yokebar www.yokebar.com

Important Tools for Exercise

- Timer that does interval times. You can use a timer to set for 1 minute times, but it becomes a little cumbersome to constantly start. Since you have to start the time it is easy to cheat. www. gymboss.com

- Timer to set for the entire session goal

- Water

- Great Music

Exercises for Interval Training

Hi5 Health System

FOOD & FUEL
- Cut meal size in 1/2
- Choose low glycemic foods
- No calorie counting
- Balance pH & alkalotic foods
- Photo each meal

~ Daily Routine ~

High Nutrient drink
H₂O
Fruit
Fiber
Enzyme
Probiotics
EFA
Vit/Min

MEALS: 5 meals per day

Breakfast
Snack
Lunch
Snack
Dinner

Energy Foods that fuel

* Back-up plan!!
* Triple Threat: 50/50 lunges, 50 p/u, 100 abs

www.hi5healthnetwork.com

Warning! Highly processed white bread, white pasta, white sweeteners, soft drinks and high fructose corn syrup ARE TOXIC!

FITNESS!

Exercise is a gift! Proven to decrease all forms of disease, slow down the aging process, eliminate depression, balance hormones and improve all aspects of life!

WHAT DO YOU LIKE TO DO?

Plan ahead, keep it simple & be consistent. 10-25 min/day.

Week 1:
Week 2:
Week 3:
Week 4:
Week 5:

Family
YOUR WHY!!

Everyone is standing for attention. Give it freely. Tell them daily!

What will you do?

FUN!

Hang out with happy people!

What will you do to fun this week?

Be Optimistic!

Faith

Your life has   Find the peace to   Ask for your

What will you do this week to grow your faith?

Hi5 Health System

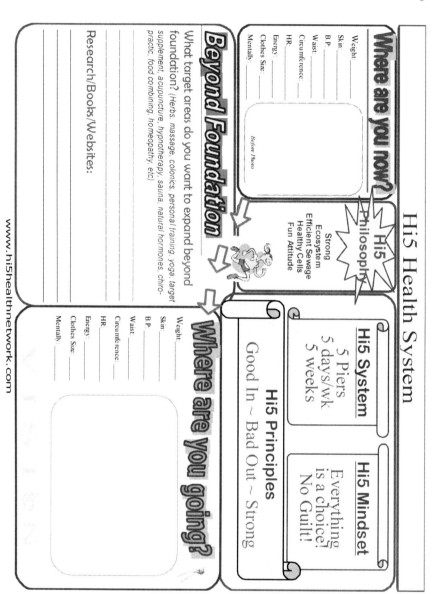

Where are you now?

Weight:
Skin:
B.P:
Waist:
Circumference:
HR:
Energy:
Clothes Size:
Mentally:

Before Photo

Hi5 Philosophy

Strong
Ecosystem
Efficient Sewage
Healthy Cells
Fun Attitude

Hi5 System

5 Piers
5 days/s/wk
5 weeks

Hi5 Mindset

Everything
is a choice!
No Guilt!

Hi5 Principles

Good In ~ Bad Out ~ Strong

Beyond Foundation

What target areas do you want to expand beyond foundation? (Herbs, massage, colonics, personal training, yoga, target supplement, acupuncture, hypnotherapy, sauna, natural hormones, chiropractic, food combining, homeopathy, etc)

Research/Books/Websites:

Where are you going?

Weight:
Skin:
B.P:
Waist:
Circumference:
HR:
Energy:
Clothes Size:
Mentally:

BONUS

Affirmations to print and post

I AM GREAT, I AM THE BEST, I AM STRONG, I AM MEN-
TALLY CAPABLE, I AM PHYSICALLY CAPABLE, I AM SPIRI-
TUALLY CAPABLE, THERE IS NO WALL THAT CAN KEEP
ME FROM REACHING MY GOAL, MY LIMIT, THE TOP.....
TILL FOREVER, I HAVE NOTHIN' TO WORRY ABOUT BE-
CAUSE I KNOW THAT GOD IS RIGHT THERE......REPEAT!!!!!
REPEAT!!!! REPEAT!!!!

*"now i know that this is a lot to say and i know that your gap(free time) is basi-
cally filled, but this is for anything so i suggest that you save it."*

author
Ariana Locsin 12 years old

Visit www.hi5healthnetwork.com for more affirmations and ideas for
reprogramming your self talk.

CPSIA information can be obtained at www.ICGtesting.com
Printed in the USA
LVOW030659181111

255412LV00003BA/2/P